Treat 12 Types of Cancer Using Graviola/Sours

op

1. Introduction

Nature is generous and it does not stop surprising us and amaze us through the products it delivers us. The soursop fruit and leaves have always been used to cure many pathologies. A few years ago, American and Korean researchers have argued that with this tropical fruit, we can overcome the evil of the century that is cancer. Is it true ? Let us enumerate here what brings us this miraculous fruit.

It is an exotic small tree 3 to 10 meters high that the indigenous populations of the Caribbean, Central America, South, and Amazon know well to make a traditional medicinal use. Called soursop, graviola, sapodilla or guanabana depending on the country, one and the same plant hides behind these names: the Annona muricata, family Annonaceae. All parts of the tree are used: leaves, root flowers, seeds, fruits, bark. Very popular, the white pulp of its big fruits bristling with excrescences, with the taste of lychee, is consumed in the form of fruit juice, smoothie, donuts or sorbet. Rich in vitamin C, fiber, iron, potassium, calcium, amino acids and various alkaloids, it is given many virtues: diuretic, galactologue (promotes lactation), antipyretic (fight against fever) antidiarrheal and antiparasitic, antiarthritic ... Infusions and decoctions of its leaves, flowers, roots and bark, are known as calming, fighting against insomnia, headaches, hypertension, diabetes and asthma. As for seeds, they also have antiparasitic and insecticidal properties ...

Since the dawn of time, this sweet and sweet and sour fruit is used in traditional medicine to relieve pain and prevent many pathologies.

The taste of the soursop fruit is slightly sour and its flavor is described as a combination of pineapple and strawberry flavor. Its skin is thorny, but its flesh is juicy and delicious. Further studies are needed to prove the benefits of corossol cancer, but the limited consumption of soursop is not harmful to health, cancer patients can consume soursop regularly and can benefit from its health benefits. The seeds are not edible, but the fruit pulp has several medicinal properties.

2. Medicinal benefits of soursop.

The fibrous flesh of soursop helps to improve digestive health. Cancer patients suffer from several problems of the digestive system such as constipation, indigestion, because of strong drugs, chemotherapy drugs, etc. These problems can be naturally relieved by the consumption of fibrous fruits.

Experts believe that soursop can heal cancer (if it is detected at the earliest). Soursop supplements are also available on the market. The benefits of Corossol against cancer include the destruction of cancer cells without damaging healthy cells. So, it can be a good alternative to chemotherapy. But as long as these properties are not scientifically proven, we can not accept them as facts. However, the consumption of soursop fruit can certainly be useful for patients with cancer. But excessive consumption should be avoided.

With soursop fruits, bark, leaves and soursop tree roots are commonly used as ingredients with various traditional medicinal herbs. Soursop leaves help calm the nerves. Tea prepared with soursop leaves works as an analgesic. The sap of its leaves, or flesh, can be applied locally to get rid of eczema, rashes and swelling. Topical application promotes rapid healing of wounds and prevents infections.

Cancer and cancer treatment like chemotherapy results in weak immune system. Patients are more likely to catch infections. Vitamin C in soursop is an antioxidant vitamin that helps strengthen the immune system and helps prevent infections like urinary tract infections, coughs and colds.

3. Results of chemotherapy in the low number of globules

Corossol gives iron and thus, can improve the number of red blood cells. It also contains riboflavin, which helps relieve headaches. Soursop thiamine helps boost energy levels. Cooper in soursop helps maintain healthy bones by promoting the absorption of calcium from ingested foods.

Soursop juice works very well for liver problems. It is believed that this can reduce inflammation of the urethra and therefore, can reduce symptoms such as pain when urinating.

Corossol tea is used to treat gall bladder disease. The extract obtained from the leaves and stems could be effective in destroying cancer cells. In addition, the consumption of soursop can be beneficial because it has no side effects (when consumed in limited quantities).

Some reports from the study show that the chemical found in soursop is almost 10,000 times more potent than Adriamycin, the drug used in chemotherapy, and so it may be beneficial if it is used to kill cells; cancerous colon (without causing damage to healthy cells).

Studies show that soursop is beneficial in treating nearly twelve different types of cancer, including the most common cancers such as colon, breast, lung, pancreatic cancer and prostate cancer. It has also been noticed that the immune system of cancer patients who have consumed during soursop chemotherapy cycles has not been impaired or weakened much, compared to other cancer patients. Browse through another soursop item and cure cancer for more information.

Since Soursop is high in sugar, it must be consumed in limited quantities. Cancer patients can consume soursop and enjoy its health benefits with chemotherapy. Corossol can at least reduce the side effects of chemotherapy. And if it kills the cancer cells naturally, then that's fine. Cancer patients are advised to consult an oncologist or health care provider before opting for soursop. The doctor will explain how much soursop would be enough to reap the health benefits.

4. Soursop and its medicinal properties

Thanks to its multiple components, soursop helps fight against many pathologies. Ever since, fruits, leaves, barks and roots of graviola are used as a preventive and curative to relieve pain and fight against diseases like insomnia, different kinds of infection, various types of inflammations as well as wounds and diseases of the skin.

Here is a non-exhaustive list:

- cases of insomnia, depression and nervous disorders,

- bacterial, parasitic and fungal infections,

- cardiac pathology and digestive problem,

- constipation, intestinal colic, diarrhea, dysentery,

- liver problems,

- Arthritis,

- bronchial abscess,

- edema, ringworm, herpes,

- malaria.

In addition, soursop and its derivatives are very effective as analgesic, tranquilizer and antispasmodic.

5. Benefits of Soursop for health

The fibrous flesh of soursop helps to improve digestive health. Cancer patients suffer from several problems of the digestive system such as constipation, indigestion, because of strong drugs, chemotherapy drugs, etc. These problems can be naturally relieved by the consumption of fibrous fruits.

Experts believe that soursop can heal cancer (if it is detected at the earliest). Soursop supplements are also available on the market. The benefits of Corossol against cancer include the destruction of cancer cells without damaging healthy cells. So, it can be a good alternative to chemotherapy. But as long as these properties are not scientifically proven, we can not accept them as facts. However, the consumption of soursop fruit can certainly be useful for patients with cancer. But excessive consumption should be avoided.

With soursop fruits, bark, leaves and soursop tree roots are commonly used as ingredients with various traditional medicinal herbs. Soursop leaves help calm the nerves. Tea prepared with soursop leaves works as an analgesic. The sap of its leaves, or flesh, can be applied locally to get rid of eczema, rashes and swelling. Topical application promotes rapid healing of wounds and prevents infections.

Cancer and cancer treatment like chemotherapy results in weak immune system. Patients are more likely to catch infections. Vitamin C in soursop is an antioxidant vitamin that helps strengthen the immune system and helps prevent infections like urinary tract infections, coughs and colds.

6. Results of chemotherapy in the low number of globules

Corossol gives iron and thus, can improve the number of red blood cells. It also contains riboflavin, which helps relieve headaches. Soursop thiamine helps boost energy levels. Cooper in soursop helps maintain healthy bones by promoting the absorption of calcium from ingested foods.

Soursop juice works very well for liver problems. It is believed that this can reduce inflammation of the urethra and therefore, can reduce symptoms such as pain when urinating.

Corossol tea is used to treat gall bladder disease. The extract obtained from the leaves and stems could be effective in destroying cancer cells. In addition, the consumption of soursop can be beneficial because it has no side effects (when consumed in limited quantities).

Some reports from the study show that the chemical found in soursop is almost 10,000 times more potent than Adriamycin, the drug used in chemotherapy, and so it may be beneficial if it is used to kill cells; cancerous colon (without causing damage to healthy cells).

Studies show that soursop is beneficial in treating nearly twelve different types of cancer, including the most common cancers such as colon, breast, lung, pancreatic cancer and prostate cancer. It has also been noticed that the immune system of cancer patients who have consumed during soursop chemotherapy cycles has not been impaired or weakened much, compared to other cancer patients. Browse through another soursop item and cure cancer for more information.

Since Soursop is high in sugar, it must be consumed in limited quantities. Cancer patients can consume soursop and enjoy its health benefits with chemotherapy. Corossol can at least reduce the side effects of chemotherapy. And if it kills the cancer cells naturally, then that's fine. Cancer patients are advised to consult an oncologist or health care provider before opting for soursop. The doctor will explain how much soursop would be enough to reap the health benefits.

7. Soursop and cancer

For several decades, Californian researchers have been studying the virtues of soursop in cases of cancer and cancerous tumors. They are still in the research phase, but they argue that soursop extract is a powerful antioxidant, that it boosts the immune system, acts effectively on cancer cells without damaging healthy ones, and is able to replace chemotherapy.

The action of soursop is 10,000 times superior to that of adriamycin, a drug used in chemotherapy. So be patient and wait to see the results of this research so promising. Nothing prevents us from now to consume at will soursop and to take advantage of the benefits of its leaves, barks and roots.

8. Efficiency in the study

Virtually unknown in the West, soursop has acquired in recent years, thanks to the Internet and social networks, a solid reputation as an anti-cancer plant. The articles abound, in French and especially in English, where the plant is called under its name of graviola. The arguments put forward, far from being always substantiated, point to the extraordinary anti-tumor activity of corossol, capable of neutralizing malignant cells. Sometimes, conclusive clinical studies - carried out on the human being - are evoked ... Some sites relaying this information, of a very unequal quality, promote the plant, by selling dry extracts of its leaves in the form of capsules ... Still others claim that the extraordinary discoveries concerning soursop, known for several years, have been hidden by the pharmaceutical industry, which, in the impossibility of patenting the living or synthesizing the assets of the plant, would seek to protect its financial monopoly on chemotherapy treatments ... Prudence therefore, and especially in case of evocation of the conspiracy theory, because one can wonder what credit to give to these massive and unanimous affirmations of anti-cancer miracle plant.

9. A hundred studies on Soursop

One thing is certain: soursop has been the subject of a hundred research programs since the mid-1990s in the United States, India, Japan, Korea and Europe, including France. In vitro and in vivo studies, published in scientific journals, have demonstrated its antimicrobial, antiviral (especially against herpes HSV-1 and HSV-2), anti-inflammatory (especially against arthritis), antidiabetic, antihypertensive (it is vasodilator and widens the blood vessels), antiparasitic, insecticides, or even hepatoprotective. A comprehensive review of its virtues was published in 2015 in a meta-study conducted at the Faculty of Science in Kuala Lumpur, Malaysia *. But it is obviously on cancer that studies are concentrated the most ... In the viewfinder, the action of a family of active ingredients specific to the family of Annonaceae:

acetogenins. These natural compounds derived from soursop (and in particular from its leaves), such as annonacin, would thus be capable of inducing the apoptosis of cancer cells, that is to say their self-programmed death, by inhibiting an enzyme in particular (NADPH-oydase), involved in the synthesis of ATP, a molecule providing energy to cells via mitochondria. Deprived of its "pile", the cancer cell would thus see its proliferation thwarted ...

According to scientific studies, the leaves, bark and pulp of guanabana are able to kill the cells of 12 types of cancer, including cancer of the colon, prostate, liver, breast and pancreas.

It is a fact that guanabana pulp contains vitamins very useful for the body and its health - vitamins B1, B2, B3,

B5, B6, B9 and C, calcium, potassium, iron, sodium, magnesium, phosphorus, zinc.

That's why guanabana has a real vitamin bomb that, with regular and fair use, can make our body resistant to all kinds of diseases.

Since 2002, many Japanese studies have examined a large number of acetogenins present in a number of plant varieties. They used mice that included lung cancer cells.

One third, who was the control group, got absolutely nothing, one-third got a chemotherapy drug, and the other third got the primary Graviolaacetogenin, 10mg of the ad.

After a 14-day period, scientists found that 5 out of 6 in the control group survived and so their tumor masses were calculated. Compared to the control group, the chemotherapy collection revealed a 54.6% decrease in tumor mass.

Six mice died as a result of toxicity. On the other hand, those who consumed Graviola survived and their tumors inhibited by 57.9%. Compared to chemotherapy, these results were much larger. There were no toxicity issues.

Namely, by regulating blood sugar levels, guanabana, which is a plant from Central America, is able to cure diabetes. However, the media will never tell you.

Treating HIV, cancer and liver, kidney, prostate and thyroid problems is also one of the health benefits of this fruit.

This fruit is able to destroy cancer cells without harming healthy cells because of its cytotoxic properties. This is very important for the whole drug because chemotherapy, which is the conventional therapy against cancer, destroys both healthy and unhealthy cells.

Even if you can not believe this fact, but guanabana extract is able to eliminate cancer cells from 12 cancers. It is also considered 10,000 times more potent than the common chemotherapy drug called Adriamycin.

Many studies have been conducted on the effects of this plant. You should know that many of them have been able to show that this amazing plant is certainly one of the most effective natural cures for cancer. Try it, you will not regret it! Concentrated Guanabana can kill tumor cells from 12 unique types of malignancy, and is thought to be 10,000 times more effective than Adriamycin, which is a typical calm chemotherapy.

Unlike ordinary chemotherapy drugs, this organic product will not influence your healthy cells. There has been some criticism about the impact of soursop on malignancy since the 1970s. But most scientific studies have shown that this natural product is profoundly convincing against different tumor cells. But unfortunately, there has been little laboratory testing on this subject, in light of the fact that the pharmaceutical industry does not want society in general to realize the magical power of this organic product.

10. Effective in vitro on cancer cells

The properties of acetogenins have been studied in particular by Jerry L. McLaughlin of the Pharmacy and Chemistry Laboratory at Purdue University, Indiana, a research facility supported by the US National Cancer Institute. The scientist says, in a 1996 study published in the Journal of Natural Products, that some Corossol acetogenins are "10,000 times more potent" in colon cancer cells than adriamycin, a product commonly used in cancer chemotherapy * *. An astonishing discovery to support the "miraculous" nature of the plant, but it should be nuanced ... In another study conducted by the same scientist the same year, the effectiveness of other acetogens was much less spectacular , and "only" equivalent or slightly superior to the same chemotherapy product ... Anyway, many studies have demonstrated anti-tumor action, both in vitro on cancer cell lines, and in vivo, on mice grafted with tumors. This property concerns several types of cancer, lung, breast, pancreas, liver or prostate. In addition, it has been shown in the laboratory that acetogenins are selective, and only attack cancer cells, sparing healthy cells. For all that, must we cry out for the absolute cure for cancer? Certainly, no. Because, as the official body Cancer Research UK has pointed out on its website, as well as the international journal Oncology, no research has been done so far on humans ... In the absence of clinical studies, only able to assess the real effectiveness of a potentially anticancer substance, caution remains in place. This is all the more important because excessive consumption of soursop is suspected of causing nervous disorders.

While the miraculous benefits of soursop in the treatment of cancer have been scientifically proven, they seem to hide the other healing properties of this spiny fruit. Thanks to its rich components formed among other amino acids, vitamins and minerals, the Annona muricata is an all-natural therapeutic ally and certainly does not produce unexpected side effects provided you consume it with some moderation.

In fruit juice, sherbet or jam, soursop is recommended in cases of insomnia, depression and nervous disorders. It is also an antimicrobial agent for bacterial, parasitic and fungal infections. It is also good for the heart and stimulates digestion.

Originally from Amazonia, the soursop is green and vaguely resembles a heart. It is recognized that it reaches maturity by its penetrating odor and its rather soft skin.

10.   A powerful anti-cancer

Nature surprises us more and more. The virtues of this fruit are unknown by the majority of the population in the world and especially by people who have cancer. However, soursop, still known as Graviola or Guanabana, is a fruit whose anti-cancer properties are scientifically proven.

The bark, fruits, leaves and roots act on the cells of our body. The leaves of the tree can destroy the cancer cells and act ten thousand times more than the chemotherapy without any side effects (weight loss, hair loss, etc.). Graviola assures its reputation among researchers in the healing of breast, intestines, ovaries, liver and lung cancer.

All parts of this tree are used in natural medicine, nothing is lost since the bark, roots, fruits, leaves and seeds are all beneficial to the health of the human being.

According to the research results of the American University PURDUE, it is the leaves of this tree that are more important. Indeed, they can destroy cancer cells.

Its main virtue is in its active ingredient, acetogenin, which helps to selectively inhibit the growth of cancer cells. Numerous studies have established a high effectiveness of

Corossol in the reduction of tumor cells in various types of cancer.

The alkaloids present in the bark and leaves of this plant have a possible cytotoxic effect, which can be used to treat various types of malignant tumors, without attacking healthy cells. In addition it contains proteins, carbohydrates, fibers, ashes, calcium, phosphorus, iron, thiamine, riboflavin, niacin, ascorbic acid, amino acids, alkaloids and triterpenes.

It helps to strengthen the immunological system. It is recommended in the treatment of diarrhea, dysentery and other gastrointestinal ailments. It is also used in cases of nervous tension, stress and insomnia.

Graviola / Corossol (leaf powder)

Soursop is one of those trees, which is included in the list of herbal medicines, as a cure for several ailments. While ripe fruit and soursop juice. It is said to cure urethritis, the sap of its leaves is applied topically to treat eruptions of eczema and swelling. Even the flesh of this fruit is applied to the wounds, for faster healing. Soursop is also fruit used to treat certain diseases of the liver, leprosy, etc. Soursop tea is used to get rid of head lice and in the treatment of gall bladder disease. In some areas, the bark of soursop roots is used as an antidote in some forms of poisoning. Learn more about graviola extract, as Soursop is known in Portuguese.

It was during the 1970s that soursop earned a lot of publicity, as some studies suggested the possible role of soursop for cancer cures. From this period, various studies have been conducted on the connection between soursop and cancer. According to a 1976 study conducted by the National Cancer Institute, the extract derived from the leaves and stems of soursop can be effective in attacking and destroying cancer cells. After that, various studies were conducted on this topic and they came up with different positive suggestions about soursop and cure cancer. It has been suggested that the active ingredients on soursop extract target malignant cells and not those that are healthy. This avoids the side effects of chemotherapy, such as, hair loss, weight loss, etc. It has also been suggested that soursop can be more beneficial than chemotherapy, in the treatment of certain types of cancer, such as, that of colon, breast, prostate, lung, pancreas, liver, etc. A study conducted by the National University of Colombia states that the soursop fruit is very effective in the treatment of cancer.

The soursop fruit has been studied and developed as raw materials for cancer drugs, particularly cancer of the prostate, pancreas and lung. A US company willing to pay billions of dollars to prove the effectiveness of soursop as an effective cancer cell killer and a lot safer than chemotherapy. Unfortunately, so far the drug is still a secret.News about the soursop secret and was later spread quickly revealed by the mailing list. This information is quite encouraging Certainly, ESPECIALLY for people with cancer and their families. "Thank God, that's right, my father and even less eat soursop, do not have to splurge a lot of money Said Emmy, whose father was sentenced to seven months ago for lung cancer.

Currently, the number of cancer survivors is growing, and yet there is one solution that is considered to have the minimum of side effects. Although the discovery was mentioned, a soursop medicine has benefited 10 thousand times stronger than chemotherapy. In the middle of this, an American company that has long been research and development of soursop fruit (soursop) as a cure for cancer is still a secret meeting to close this miracle fruit.

11.   What exactly happens in organic soursop?

Ten thousand times more powerful. All this came from research at Purdue University, in the United States, the WHO turned out the soursop fruit is effective at killing cancer cells. Unfortunately, the results could not be communicated to the public.It seems They want to take advantage of these results. Naturally, the amount spent for research was considered very very big. Speaking of the size of soursop or graviola fruit, in fact, has long been reported research institutions in the United States. Health Sciences Institute, USA, in early 2000 revealed that the Spanish called the graviola fruit has the natural ability as a killer of cancer cells, even up to 10 thousand times stronger than that of chemotherapy uses chemicals In addition to curing cancer, soursop fruit also acts as an antibacterial, antifungal and effective agent against different types of parasites or worms. Soursop is also effective in lowering blood pressure, depression, stress, and normalizing the nervous system are interrupted. Health Sciences Research Institute taken based on the habits of Indians living in the Amazon jungle OMS.

12.   Benefits of organic soursop

Also analgesic, sedative and antispasmodic Guanábana cleanses the body. Many pharmaceutical studies have tried to synthesize the active products but without success.

Perhaps this is why no anti-cancer treatment is offered based on Soursop because laboratories can not patent a tree or a plant. Will the tropical forest and its corossolier come to revolutionize the anti-cancer therapeutics? Nothing is less economically safe.

Nothing is lost since the bark, roots, fruits, leaves and seeds are all beneficial for the health of the human being.

People have always used the fruit of this tree in cooking to make juice or ice cream.

But according to research results of the American University "Purdue", it is the leaves of this tree that are more important. Indeed, these leaves can destroy cancer cells. And it is even said that it is ten thousand times more powerful than chemotherapy.

Graviola is known to have the healing properties of breast cancer, ovaries, prostate gut, liver and lungs.

So, as it is summer, if you happen to make natural juice at home, choose the soursop juice first, it will help prevent a possible cancer but it will also help you in digestion.

You do not need to get cancer to eat this tasty fruit. So do not hesitate if you are lucky to buy some.

If the miraculous benefits of soursop in the treatment of cancer are very popular, do not obscure the other healing properties of this fruit. Indeed, thanks to its rich components, soursop is an all natural therapeutic ally. It is indicated among other things in case of insomnia and allows to have a calm and restful sleep. Soursop is also recommended for people who are anxious or stressed because the fruit fights against depression and nervous disorders.

Soursop is also recommended in case of viral infection. Thanks to the different substances it contains, soursop is able to stimulate digestion, and to fill the deficiencies in vitamins. Among other things, he treats rheumatism, arthritis and diabetes. It is also advisable for people prone to heart problems. Note that soursop is an antimicrobial agent for bacterial, parasitic and fungal infections.

The active ingredients are mostly in the leaves and seeds. While waiting for our cancers, insomnia or other ailments to be treated by the Guanábana, I propose you a refreshing recipe:

13.   COROSSOL SORBET

Ingredients:

- 50 cl of soursop juice

- 1 zest of lemon

- 1 spoon of vanilla essence

- 2 pinches of cinnamon

- 200 g caster sugar

Mix soursop juice with lemon zest, vanilla essence, cinnamon and caster sugar. Beat vigorously and pour into a pan. Ice in an ice cream maker preferably for 3 hours. It's ready, treat yourself! In Costa Rica, on the markets, there is always a street vendor offering glasses of this nectar for 300 colones glass. To taste without waiting ...

Some parts of the tree, such as bark, roots, leaves, fruit pulp and seeds, have been used for centuries as medicine by tribal people. Graviola or soursop believed to be the

Amazon as a heart to cure diseases, asthma, liver failure (liver), and rheumatism.The National Cancer Institute has conducted research on graviola since 1976. The trial was conducted in 20 different independent laboratories under the supervision of the National Cancer Institute.Only chasing the evilIn Asia, a similar study conducted in South Korea. A study published in the Journal of Natural Products States, a study conducted at the Catholic University of South Korea stated that one of the announced acetogenin chemicals named named graviola, capable of selecting, distinguishing, and killing cells cancerous ones develop in the colon that.

What are the most spectacular discoveries of the study?

The anticancer agent has also been able to select and kill only the malignant cancer cells, while intact healthy cells. Compare with chemotherapy, the. Which has been used to treat cancer patients can not distinguish between cancer cells and healthy WHO cells. Reproductive cells (such as the stomach and hair) have been killed in chemotherapy. Impact, the negative effects arising from the form of nausea, hair loss, and drastic weight loss.In addition, the effectiveness of soursop fruit is to protect the immune system and prevent deadly infections. Implications for cancer patients is their increased energy and improved physical appearance.

14.   Boiled leaves

In Indonesia, soursop as a natural remedy has also long been recognized. Dose never tried herbal therapists to deal with the growth of cancer cells is 10 soursop have dark green leaves with 3 cups of boiling water (600 cc), and is left in the pay of a cup of water (200 cc). Once cooled, then filtered and drank the water every morning (there are those who drink patients early in the afternoon).

Effect of decoction consumption of soursop leaves is the stomach feels warm or warm, and then the body will sweat profusely. It must be understood that the use of powerful herbal ingredients are not directly or immediately recovered alias cespleng that the effects of chemical drugs has to offer. That is, it took discipline to drink a potion for 3-4 weeks.After that, new effects can be felt and even then, it can not be scientifically tested, rely more on empirical evidence or admiralty.Hambali (33 years old) prostate cancer patients admitted, after soda juice drink diligent sugar-free in a better state. Could he go back to work after a hard move? If examined in the laboratory, it turns out that the cancer cells to dry. As other cells grow (hair, nails, etc.) has not been disturbed. Given the effectiveness of these, it would be wonderful if the results of scientific research could be the basis of knowledge of the public and use soursop as a cancer drug, to give a glimmer of hope to people with this deadly disease.

The infusion of the leaves is calming and promotes digestion

The leaves, macerated in warm water, can be used as a poultice to relieve burns caused by sunburn. They are also used for the preparation of calming baths for infants.

- The leaves and bark are sedative in the form of lukewarm infusion.

Against strong emotions, to calm the nerves, take seven leaves and a finger of bark that you throw in a liter of boiling water.

To fight against insomnia, take a sweet brew of three to six leaves for a cup of water before going to bed.

- Against the irritation of the intestines, macerate in one or two liters of water a small green soursop, cut into small pieces. After one hour of maceration, consume the drink obtained.

- Against the lymphangitis, apply on the sick part a ripe fruit crushed and sprinkled with camphorated alcohol.

15. Drinking soursop leaf ragout

I want to share your experiences of eating boiled soursop leaves to fight prostate metastases and bone cancer that I have suffered. About prostate cancer itself can be read in stage 4 prostate cancer. Since known to suffer from prostate cancer and bone metastases 10 months ago I tried to get to other non-medical treatment in addition to the medical treatment that I lead. Armed with an internet search and experience I received from some other cancer patients then I decided to eat boiled leaves of soursop juice soursop and herbal therapies in addition to to satisfy the needs lainnya.Untuk corossol leaves so I decided to buy soursop trees places such as posters, Mekarsari, and the seller other plant, and now at home, I had 12 soursop trees, and even so, still not enough, so I took soursop leaves from a neighbor who happens to have a soursop tree.The ways to make decoction of soursop leaves can be read on the internet, and I consume on a decoction regular soursop leaves 2 cups a day until now.

In accordance with the description of the demo below for soursop leaves boiling in Taman Blooms Sari fruit in February 2011, then the decoction of soursop leaves should not be stored beyond 12 hours I tried the stew is stored more than 12 hours was already stale and creates a feeling of not consuming, I enak.Untuk soursop juice without sugar and after the Sari Bloom wish to be informed whether it should be given to palm sugar excellence instead granulated sugar. The effects of drinking sopped soursop leaves are that the body feels a bit warmer.

Since the last 3 months of medical treatment I have experienced hormonal suspension by a doctor and only monitored the PSA (for the prostate tumor marker) not to exceed> 4, and since 3 months ago, I was much more dependent on decoction of soursop / soursop juice compared to other herbal medicine. The changes that I feel now is the growth of black hair strokes on the head when my family has had a hereditary problem with gray hair is relatively young age, to myself since the age of 50 are no longer the black hair strokes on the head. I just realized the existence of black hair, after a meeting with a friend who said head hair look more black.Me, I do not know if it is in reaction to consume leaves soursop, the clearer when we read the literature on the leaves of soursop the soursop have said that the effect a thousand times that chemotherapy and unlike chemotherapy that it has the benefits of soursop leaf cells only kill the bad cells alone. Are soursop leaves the drink is also regularly relive a dead SEL2, Wallahualam. Certainly, which adds to my belief that soursop cooking leaves a positive effect in the fight against cancer and PSA pengechekan Mudah2an at least 2 weeks, I was able to maintain a PSA rate

Most people who develop cancer are due to how they eat and what they eat. Bad foods, create an internal ground that has allowed the body to be filled with fungi (eg tobacco leaves are filled with mushrooms, as well as peanuts, to name just two of the many substances commonly consumed) , so that when a carcinogen reacted with the body, the internal ground could not deal with the carcinogen and the person had cancer. So, by default, if you want to get back on your cancer, you have to go back to your diet to create a strong inner terrain.

Graviola, a powerful antioxidant, can help you combat this plague and revise your diet to regain a much better health.

How many people have died while this billion-dollar drug maker has concealed the secret of the miraculous soursop tree! This small tree is called graviola in Brazil, Guanabara in Spanish and "soursop" in English. The fruit may be large and the juice acid and the sweet white pulp is eaten or, more commonly, it is made of fruit drinks, sorbets, etc.

The main interest of this plant is in its strong anti-carcinogenic effect.

Although it is as effective for many other medical conditions, it is its antitumor effect that is of greatest interest. This plant is a cure for cancer, proven for various types of cancers. In addition to being a cure for cancer, the soursop has a wide range of antimicrobial agents for bacterial and fungal infections, it is effective against parasites and intestinal worms, hypertension, and depression. In addition, it reduces nervous disorders.

If there is one argument that sheds light on this, it is the fact that in America many health science institutes are aware of the incredible history of the soursop tree.

The truth is surprisingly simple: hidden deep in the Amazon!

The rainforest has produced a tree that could literally revolutionize our medicine; and the rest of the world is looking for cancer treatment by chance, survival ... The future has never been so much a promoter of hope for a cure for cancer.

The research done with the extracts of this miraculous tree is now possible, and the expected benefits are considerable:

-Combat cancer, without accident, and effectively with an all natural therapy that no longer causes nausea, weight loss, hair loss, ...

- Protect your immune system and prevent deadly infections

- Allow the patient to feel stronger and healthier during treatment

-Increase your energy and improve your life expectancy...!

The source of this information is stunning: it comes from America (the largest manufacturers of remedies), the fruit of more than 20 laboratory tests conducted since the 1970s!

Extracts from the tree showed that:

* Effectively, they kill the target and kill the malignant cells in 12 types of cancer, including "colon", breast, prostate, lung and pancreatic cancer. ....

- The compounds of the tree have been shown up to 10,000 times stronger to slow the growth of cancer cells than Adriamycin, a chemotherapy drug commonly used!

- Even though it is more effective than chemotherapy, the compound extracted from selectivelyhunts from the soursop tree only kills cancer cells; it does not harm healthy cells!

The amazing anti-carcinogenic properties of the soursop tree have been considerably proven - if the soursop extract is as promising as it looks, - why would not every doctor oncologist use it on all his patients?

The answer cools and illustrates just how easily our health - and for many, our very lives (!) - are controlled by money and power. The soursop tree - the plant that is grown in America "the largest drug makers with billions of dollars" have started a search for a cure for cancer, and their research has been focused on the soursop tree, a legendary healing tree from the Amazon Rainforest.

The various parts of the soursop tree - including bark, leaves, roots, fruit, and fruit-seeds - have been used for centuries by healing wizards and native Indians of North America. South to treat heart disease, asthma, liver problems and arthritis.

Continue the very little documented scientific evidence: the company paid money and resources into testing the properties of the anti-cancer tree - and they were shocked by the results: The soursop tree is revealed as a dynamo destroying cancer. But, where the history of the soursop tree almost ended, it is when the company stumbled on a serious problem concerning this tree: - the product is completely natural and, according to the federal law, non-patentable. It was therefore not possible to make any serious profits.

Thus, the medicine company invested almost seven years, trying to synthesize two substances of the tree, anti-carcinogenic ingredients of the most powerful. If they had managed to isolate them, they could have produced clones made by humans, and thus hold the power of the tree. Then they could have patented it to get a profit on their money invested...

Alas, they have erred in vain; the original substance can not be easily reproduced.

So there was no way for the company to protect its profits - or even the brand of the drug that would offset the millions paid in research.

As the dream of huge profits vanished, their experiences on the tree also stopped. And worse, the company even abandoned the entire project and chose not to publish the conclusions of his research!

Fortunately, there was a scientist from the tree research team, whose conscience would not tolerate such an atrocity. Risking his career, he contacted a company that was committed to harvesting the medicinal plants of the Amazon rainforest, and kicked off...! The miracle began when researchers at the Institute of Health Sciences were alerted to the importance of the soursop tree. They began to focus their research on "the deadly tree of cancer."

Evidence of the amazing effectiveness of the Soursop tree, and its outrageous camouflage operation, was quickly found.

The National Cancer Institute carried out the first scientific research in 1976. The results showed that the soursop tree "leaves and stems were found effective in combating destructive malignant cells".

Inexplicably, the results were published in an internal report never exposed to the public...

-Since 1976, the soursop tree has proven to be an extremely powerful cancer killer in 20 independent laboratory tests; yet no clinical trial has taken place - physicians knowledgeable about the main point of view, typical references and journals used to judge the value of a treatment - nothing has ever been done ....

-An article published in the Journal of Natural Products, according to a recent study by the Catholic University of South Korea, indicated that a chemical capable of killing colon cancer cells was found in soursop. The said product has 10,000 times the power of Adriamycin (usually used chemotherapy remedy).

-The most significant part of this study from the Catholic University of South Korea is that Soursop attacks only the carcinogenic cells, leaving the healthy cells intact.

Chemotherapy, on the contrary, indiscriminately attacks all active reproductive cells (such as the cells of the stomach and hair), causing often devastating side effects such as: nausea, and hair loss in cancer patients etc.

A study at Purdue University recently found that the leaves of the soursop tree selectively killed cancer cells, among six categories of human cells and were especially effective against the prostate, pancreatic cancer and lung cancer.

Healthful way back to a healthy state

2) The fruit contains a substance called acetogenin that has been proven to be 10,000 (ten thousand times) stronger than acetogenin, the drug used for chemo treatment worldwide with the result of 90% to 10% alone survivors - a Bingo game with the lives of people in all nations

because healing is already known.

3) As it is a nutrient it works inside out - eating cancer cells, any type of virus, bacteria nutrients, etc. do not have any side effects on our body! - Amazing, miraculous, but it's true (I had the honor of experiencing many people with cancer even in a very advanced state who were getting well with a juice containing Graviola and there is 1000 in Latin America who had the chance to know about it for 9 years of applications.Solution, Cure real and permanently cure without chemo.In the event that doctors order Chemo this special prepared juice has the powers to protect healthy cells from burning and only allows cancer cells to be destroyed, no nausea, no hair loss, nor other common side effects taking this powerhouse of healing at the same time.

My mother would not be alive without Graviola.

It's time to share and shake the world of cancer and move

from 90% to 10% in 10% to 90% of survivors!

Here is the chance to learn about a fact that there is something that has the power to cure cancer, that it has been scientifically proven and that it has been hidden away from people because it comes from Mother Nature and cannot be patented in any way.

General information: About the factory:

Graviola is an evergreen tree growing in the Amazon region of Brazil and in other countries that are affected by the Amazon rainforest. It also grows in the rainforest of North America. It grows to 15 meters tall covered with green, long and shiny leaves. Its divine fruit is green, sometimes a little bright yellow, has the shape of a human heart with a kind of skin resembling a large cactus. Its white flesh is edible fruit and people can buy it at local markets. The diameter of the fruit is 20 to 40 cm and the local people are eating it by hand, the dough is used to produce a refreshing sour-acid drink or sorbet.

Indian tribes use Graviola as medicine for centuries

Graviola has a very long history in natural herbal tribal medicine. There are healing substances in all parts of the plant: part of the powerful effects of the fruit we find high effective substances in the leaves, roots, trunk, bark and seeds. Indian tribes know the value of this miraculous tree and they use different parts of Tor multiple and varied diseases and health imbalances. Some examples:

In Roots of Brazil, the trunk and leaves are used as a sedative and tee against nervousness, in other Latin American countries as a sedative and as an average heart tonic, also for diabetes. The leave tee is also used for leverage problems and mixed with olive oil, it is used for rheumatism, arthritis and osteoarthritis pain in Peru. In Brazil they prepare a mixture from an immature fruit mixed with olive oil as a treatment against extern Arthritis and Rheumatism.

The leaves are also used against parasites in Brazil and Peru against catarrh.

Fruits, seeds and leaves are applied against fever, all kinds of parasites, worms, diarrhea, in Brazil also to help increase women's milk after childbirth.

In other countries like Haiti, the West Indies and Jamaica are Graviola using as anti spasmodic, sedative, cough and flu, like te nerve strengthening, asthma, hypertension and all kinds of parasites, the diarrhea and problems during childbirth.

Graviola and Science -Cancer Research - Scientific Results on Graviola

The Graviola fruit is already being researched since the late 19th century - At that time, science discovered that the plant has components, natural principles and properties called "Annonacaeous acetogenins", the natural chemicals that are confirmed to be very effective against many types of tumor cells with components that are found to be toxins that kill cancer cells in a very specific way. Simply speaking Graviola has elements that are able to isolate each cancer cell, build a kind of bubble around it to prevent the cancer cell can get all the nutrients away, it dies. Dead cancer cells are eliminated by the body's own system without any side effects. These components are hidden in all parts of the tree and in different combinations they are used for many different types of the disease. They are documented as anti-microbus, anti-parasitic, antitumor, anti-cancer, anti-depressive and anti-spasmodic. Several results of the study have been published, but few people have responded.

Since 1976, extensive research by the National Cancer Institute of the United States has resulted in the healing of a large intestine "adenocarcinoma" after a short time. The therapeutic effect confirmed the power of Graviola and its components. This powerful component was discovered by the German researcher and oncologist Helmut Keller and with more than three scientists they have carried out numerous studies on Graviola. Since the plant does not allow chemical processes without losing the healing powers, no one ever comes to know of this effective treatment for cancer. WHY??? - Because it only works in its natural form and a plant cannot be patented, in any form, so that the pharmaceutical world and monopolies could not get any profit and that is the reason why they hided information.

Result

Graviola contains very active, cytotoxic effects against cancer cells with a chemo therapeutic potency that is 10,000 x stronger than Adriamicin, the drug that is used for traditional chemotherapy, - without any kind of side effects!

(For a while, the HSI now offers copies of the results that can be purchased for 25.00 USD)

After confirming that Graviola can naturally cure cancer the National Health Institute has reported 20 labs to factory studies for 20 years without any results to turn the active ingredients into a worthwhile remedy. In the end they gave up and left the miraculous results in the drawer of their institutes.

Since 1996, other groups of scientists have been researching Graviola and found that the fruit has characteristics against tumor formation and that it produces selective toxins against different types of cancer cells, without attacking healthy cells. They confirmed the findings of their findings were published 8 different clinical studies.

The different studies of different laboratories leads to incredible conclusions that Graviola's Acetogenins have an unbeatable component in preventing enzyme formations, which are found in the diaphragm by tumors and cancer cells. That's why, why they are toxic only to cancer cells without attacking healthy cells. Acetonins recognize diseased cells isolates individual cancer cells and for missing nutrients the cancer cell dies.

In the year 1997, a small group of scientists discovered

that Graviola also contains alkaloids that have an anti-depressive effect. In the same year UNIVERSITY Pardu published the information that they discovered even more powers within Graviola. Their clinical studies confirmed that "Acetonin Annonacae" in Graviola are so effective that they not only kill normal cancer cells, but are also very effective at killing cancer cells that are resistant to chemotherapy. This investigation explained how this is possible: Cancer cells that survive chemotherapy have developed resistance against many other types of drugs, called Multi-Drug-Resistant (MDR) which makes them immune to any treatment and leads the patient 100% to death.

After 20 years of industry research Pharma became aware of the plant and began looking for their own research of a form and how to turn the active ingredients and components into a cure for cancer. They also failed.

Graviola does not allow any type of chemical reproduction. It is confirmed that Graviola only works as it grows in nature and beats cancer better than any synthetic drug or heavy poison rays. Until today, many different groups of scientists are still looking to create a product similar to that of Annonacins and it still works as it grew up in nature.

All that information was kept secret because Pharmacies could not turn it into something that would give them a huge profit. So, they have given proof that they are not really interested in healing people, but making huge profits from those who are already sufficiently hidden by the disease itself. Why does someone create so many unnecessary pain when there is something much stronger and without any side effects life threatening.

In the late nineties one of the scientists who was part of one of the research teams broke the silence for reasons of conscience and some of the reports were accessible to the world of medicine. Simultaneously some people from Brazil are getting away from the divine direction to go to the Amazon and study the plants of the rainforest. They have been integrating indigenous peoples to learn from them that their knowledge about healing plants of the rainforest is going back in time for many centuries.

The good thing is that for once in this world of science is not to find a way of manipulation - the healing power of cancer lies in Graviola and several other factories that God has preserved to be used as the all-purpose Powerful lets grow. It is a blessing for humanity and a gift of Mother Earth - A wake up call to become aware and begin to honor the gifts we have forgotten that they exist. When we destroy tropical forests we destroy the lungs of our planet and without oxygen any life will die. We need to open our hearts to understand that everything we experience has a solution and all we suffer from different types of the disease has a natural way of healing in nature.

Nutritional values of Graviola

minerals

Iron, potassium, calcium, copper, magnesium, manganese, sodium, phosphorus, sulfur, selenium, zinc,

vitamins

Vitamin A, vitamin B1, vitamin B2, vitamin B3, vitamin C

In addition

Dietary fiber, tannins, proteins, fat

Ethno-medicine uses Graviola in different tropical countries and USA

Latin America:

Brazil:

Abscess, tumors, edema, Worms, all kinds of parasites, bronchitis, breathing difficulties, cough, diabetes, digestive imbalances, dysentery, intestinal parasites, intestinal / colic attacks, fever, liver disorders, neuralgia, nervousness , body pain in general, rheumatism, tetanus

Peru

Tumors of all kinds, trainee ulcers, parasites, lice, diabetes Hypertension, dysentery, indigestion, inflammation, influenza, liver disorders, spasms, fever and as a sedative

Panama:

Tumors, ulcers, parasites, worms, digestive disorders (dyspepsia), diarrhea and kidney problems: Renal insufficiency - renal failure

Mexico:

Tapeworm, indigestion, diarrhea, dysentery, fever, colds,

ringworm, scurvy, styptic (bleeding)

The Caribbean:

Colds, chills, fever, flu, diarrhea, indigestion, nervousness,

palpitations, rash, spasms, skin diseases, and as a sedative

and soothing agent

Curacao:

Gallbladder problems, nervousness, as a sedative and

calming agent, childbirth

Haiti:

Parasites, lice, flu, slow digestive, diarrhea, fever, cough,

pain, weakness, injury, pellagra, nervousness, heart

disease, spasm, sedative helps with lactation, after

childbirth,

Jamaica:

Pests, Worms, asthma, fevers, heart disease, hypertension,

helps with breastfeeding after childbirth, nervousness,

sedative, spasms, tetanus, fluid retention and general weakness,

Trinity:

Ringworms, blood cleansing agent, hypertension, palpitations, syncope, insomnia, postpartum lactation help, flu,

United States:

Cancer, tumors, ulcers, fungal infections, intestinal hypertension parasites, depression

Asia - Malaysia

Boils, coughs, colds, diarrhea, dermatoses, hypertension, rheumatism and to reduce bleeding

British West Indies:

Tumors, gut parasites, asthma, childbirth, lactation help, hypertension

Other countries:

Cancer, kidney problems, bladder insufficiency, liver disorders, dysentery, malaria, stomach problems, ringworm, lice, parasites, childbirth, asthma, hypertension, heart disease, arthritis, scurvy and sedative

Native wisdom

After learning ethnological medicine and their advanced knowledge, we must ask ourselves who is more advanced.

They do not have hospitals and they do not have CANCER or have you ever seen an aboriginal in a department of a cancer hospital? They do not have laboratories, they do not turn a plant into a pill, and they are cured.

The natives still show us today how to live with nature and how nature offers everything we need for a healthy life.

What do we do with the so-called civilized world with nature and with oneself? We allow the destructive exploitation, the exhaustion, the exhaustive culture, the thieving economy, not only with Mother Nature, but also with our own lives. We burn the candle by both ends disrespects the sanctity of our body. We abuse the maximum and the end is a deadly disease. Is it a wonder? No, it's only the consequence of our questions, our habits, our believe that systems and our actions, thoughts, words about ability and look away when things are not in harmony with the order cosmic. We do not care when he does not hit us personally. To heal, we really have to heal all the kingdoms we live in otherwise we do not get a dynamic healing. Can you feel that? It is not a question of understanding, but of feeling!! We turned our feelings down

You go against your feelings and you get sick!

How many times a day do we do this???? We must return to the heart and stand up for the safety of natural resources that are still intact like the rainforest as the largest source of medicinal plants that exist in our world.

A German doctor went on vacation in the Amazonian region and wondered how many natural remedies are on the market. He took a part of the temptation and I started teaching in Germany on Graviola and the rainforest, he appeared and said: I am a director of a hospital and I was looking for a way to empower people Amazonian healing available. I our hospital, we have a new system and are open for alternative healing methods. We offer open seminars and you can come when you want to talk about cancer and other diseases. I did it for diabetes... it was amazing

Thus, Western countries are learning Graviola and the healing powers of Graviola, the miraculous fruit that brings endless surprises to people with cancer and other serious diseases. Graviola is a chance for all those who are hidden by cancer or any of the other diseases of civilization.

This newsletter is once again a wakeup call and a chance to survive cancer. I

Graviola is not only a miracle against cancer cells, but also has components (research results) that eliminate other chemicals such as cortisone, drugs and all kinds of poisons in our body. This is unique as cortisone remains in people's bodies forever with the terrible side effect that people gain weight comes nothing. Graviola is the power of life that is able to clean all the poisons we are exposed to today in our daily lives in the air, water and nutrients. It has the incredible natural power to cleanse and regenerate our body cells. Remember that our body is the sacred temple of life that deserves all our respect because the body gives us the gift of being alive and experiencing this wonderful personal journey on this beautiful planet, having fun and to grow in all directions when we maintain ourselves in a healthy state.

This plant and many others are a gift from the divine source and the Mother Earth preserved for our time to remember the love we must have for our divine vehicle, for us and for all life. Divine Source and Mother Earth have the means for people who have lost faith in the daily battle for survival.

This fruit has the shape of a huge heart to show you, even by its form that only the heart can heal without any form of human manipulation, pure and natural, as it is given.

A small glimpse of my own experiences:

As Multi-Dimensional Free Way Healer I learned to go directly to the cause of an illness that is created by feelings, psychic shocks and denial of heavy experiences on the heart and soul level as well as the use abusive body

of any kind. It can be karmic origin or even live on a place

that is more poisoned by electricity or the environment.

Nevertheless, we can never get sick when our defense of

the body works properly and opens the door to all that we

live. The path of cause and effect never fails, and even

incurable disease is curable by the cosmic law. I have

always been driven to the forest and I knew deep down

that some kind of cure for the physical body should exist in

this vast natural pharmacy of Mother Earth. I asked God to

get something in my hands that helps people understand

faster and faster to heal so they can learn on a large scale

and not just one by one.

7 years ago - I was about to travel to Germany and the day

before a friend of my spiritual group years ago more

suddenly went my way and she asked me when I'm going

to travel back to Germany and if I could help next time I'm

going to open a business that sells natural Amazon nutrients that are a healing food house and there is no one who speaks German well. Well, the word Amazon was hitting me like an electric shock and I just wanted the next day ... Is this the answer of my prayers that I thought. After a week, something pushed me to get in touch and I felt compelled to appeal. The representative came to present the products, 7 at that time. He started explaining all of them and I was holding the bottle of a mixture of Graviola and 6 other anti-cancer components in my hands instantly my whole body was increasing heat waves and huge sources that are transmitted: that's what you asked. Of course, I studied everything I had at and went to Germany for 9 months to get information on fighting the meanings and beliefs of curing traditional cancer.

There are so many cases I was testifying what it would be filling out books and it would have made you cry like it does with 100s of people when they hear people gathering annual stories that tell their stories of survival in the last moment - their desperation in the face of death and their families, penniless because no insurance would take the bills anymore - all the family sales they have to the safety of a beloved.

A friend of mine specializing in Brazilian plastic surgery got myeloid leukemia and the urgent need for a cell transplant - she was on a list of number 989 - I spent 4 months with her work on her and finally we were able to access to products and the company doctor said for her: You know you are in the hands of God? Yes - but nevertheless we will give it a try - you got to take 5 different products and we found a sponsor - today she has a foundation for abandoned animals - she left her wheelchair behind and she is very good!!

All of these experiences are divine by one, but I think the more people need to know about this - from mouth to mouth it's just slowing down - there are so many people suffering for nothing. The lady who became director of the German company had 5 types of cancer - 5 children - her best friend a director of a Hospital - he told her to go home and spend the last time with her children - which her art has come to an end and he is really sorry. At a friend's house came over and told her about these products - she loves life and she took a single product - after a week she was feeling stronger - her life powers came back, she felt that she could do and she said she would only give back and show to the front of her doctor and friend, when she was fine. After 6 months, she visited him at the hospital - he cried and asked what she was doing - she talked about the products and alleluia today's doctor is working in his hospital with these products too. It is not only hope there is a cure and that people must be informed!

Here is a little more evidence that I found in the different reports of the greatest firmness 100 Underground cures: "Magic bullet" cancer discovered - but he is silent giant pharmaceutical up!

10,000 times stronger than chemotherapy, without adverse side effects

DARYL S. had 12 tumors in her prostate. But he received advanced treatment that helped save his life. And ... In 3 months, his PSA dropped and the tumors disappeared

HOW? Daryl's secret was the help of an amazing tree that grows deep in the Amazon rainforest. Called Graviola, it could well be the ultimate fight against cancer. Studies by the National Cancer Institute already show that Graviola extract is 10,000 times stronger than top-notch chemotherapy drugs ...

Yet, it's incredible accuracy stalks cancer cells while sparing healthy cells completely alone! Graviola just seems to "know" the cells to kill and those to avoid. There is no nausea, no hair loss, no weight loss, no weakening of the immune system.

The news on Graviola sent a shockwave through the HSI medical network deepened. But the story behind Graviola is just as shocking.

As we have learned, this discovery has been about life-saving denied to humanity. And I'm sorry to say the reason is that someone was sitting on the search. The trail of the evidence clearly shows ...

For 7 long years, a billion dollar pharmaceutical company it covered up!

What's more, this is probably not the first time something like what happened. Here is a typical example of how modern pharmaceutical research works, and how your health is falling victim to the pursuit of money and power: It all began in the 1990s, when this well-known pharmaceutical giant started pouring money into the search for a cure for cancer ...

What gave Jacqueline the power CONQUEST OF BREAST CANCER?

JACQUELINE Breast Cancer, but she also had a huge advantage in her fight. Best of all, it works by using the army of your own natural bodies "killer cells". So, it actually makes you feel more energetic, rather than undermining your strength. Like many of these companies, they were intrigued by the healing powers of forest plants. They discovered that Graviola was used by Amazonian Indians to treat a wide range of diseases. And when they tested his powers against cancer, bingo, they discovered a revolution ...

But you can not do Megabucks any cure, unless you patent

...

And no one can patent a tree that has been around for

millions of years. So, the pharmaceutical company has

been trying for seven years to come with the man-made

duplicates. But they hit a brick wall. Try as they might,

they might not match Mother Nature. Finally, they

launched the towel ...

Okay, they are in business to make money. Very good. But

let me ask you ...

If the search files for this breakthrough were sitting on

your desk, what would you do with them? Call a news

conference? Send press releases?

At the very least, would not you all publish in a leading

medical journal? After all, more than 6 million Americans

have died of cancer in recent decades.

Think of how much could have been saved if a find like this had been available. But, instead of relying on independent researchers .... -

They locked up, put it on the shelf - AND turned off the light.

Fortunately, a brave researcher simply could not live with this decision. He spit out the piece ... and the result can prove to be more life-saving substance on the earth. More clinical trials are needed, but more than 20 studies to date have already established that ...

Graviola can clear 12 types of cancer cells, including breast, prostate, colon, lung and pancreatic tumors

Yet, unlike any chemotherapy drug, it leaves the cells healthy.

A miracle? Perhaps. Yet even today, not a pharmaceutical company we know has picked up and run with it.

WHY? For the same reason. Nobody can legally patent it.

Are you starting to see?

AMAZON TREE MIRACLE fights a lot more than cancer

Although scientific research on Graviola has focused on its

powers against cancer, the tree has been used for centuries

by tribal healers to treat an impressive number of diseases:

* Hypertension

* Influenza

* Ringworm

* Rheumatism

*Muscle spasm

*Neuralgia diarrhea

* Scurvy

* Malaria

* Insomnia

* The eruptions

* Dysentery

* Arthritis

HSI Reports

My report continues here: Cure Cures - and Lies About Conventional Treatments

A real example: In Germany, one of Dr. Hamer D.'s patients (work on psychic shocks to cure cancer) suffered from breast cancer and was asked three times at the hospital if she is Jewish and she denied - she had family members who were, but she was not. She wondered first why they asked that. The next day, another doctor appeared in his hospital room offering him some heavy treatment outside of chemotherapy and he told him that people with cancer have only 10% chance to survive but it could be the one of 10% when she would accept this incredible, expensive proposal. When she became aware of the reasons why she was asked to be Jewish and was not the same doctor, she said, sorry I can not do that because

I'm Jewish - the doctor said, oh, I did not know and leave the room, he pointed out: you will be fine anyway ... can you believe that? But it's the truth about heavy and expensive treatments and people believe chemo (90% is not what makes it) and suffer for nothing .... The lady reported the doctors and left the hospital . One thing is the big lie about cancer - the other side has the solution and is not sufficiently known yet to help people and children by avoiding as much unnecessary pain. You will become porter of the secret - in the month of May I will send a report on the plant and how to get the product the juice that saves 1000s lives since 9 years in Latin America and in 5 other countries - not to the States Apart from some of my friends, I sent the product to help them get better.

Conclusion

What can I say now that what I have to live experiences

with Graviola since 7 years - As I learned from advice how cases are set in motion that ends in heavy illness or disease chronic even AIDS is one of the biggest lies, during this year I am going to publish more reports on natural products and powers for a lot of diseases that are used by science as a good income, at place to inform about simple remedies from the inside. Graviola helps reproducing killer cells without our body which is self defense for which it develops rapidly as the body helps clean the nutrients to fight sick cells in the structure - any organ of them.

The latest studies conducted in Brazil have confirmed that the combination of products with Graviola has a component that kills the hospital virus even - it is a killer virus with no cure until today that is 1000 % lethal - we have achieved results that are amazing. Meanwhile, the component that has only been found.

We work to get information from alternative doctors and

healers. There is so much to learn and do because the biggest change that needs to be made in education. It is not easy to teach people who have been hunted in one direction to believe that they deny all other means, even if their own lives depend on it.

The reason for cancer is a psychic shock and it is not so difficult to learn about it - to recreate your life inside and use the fruits, plants and natural elements that Mother Earth is pushing for that we can do well. Let's open our hearts and minds to the Amazon rainforest and join people working backward to protect this latest wonder of an untouched ecosystem and stop the fire at 5,000 square miles each day for some people can make their profit. They kill life itself and we are the crown of creation and must honor all LIFE first and foremost as sacred !!

And do not forget: The miracles of life are there for

everyone

Blessings and the time of reflection.

Our tips for use

If you wish to embark on soursop supplementation, as a complementary preventive or curative treatment, you will find easily on the internet, in organic stores and in herbalist's shop dry or liquid extracts or dried leaves. Dosages recommended by distributors range from 1 to 2 grams per day in capsule form, or as an infusion of soursop leaves three times a day. Get advice and follow through your doctor's herbal practitioner. Another solution to get soursop, cheaper and simpler: you can try to grow the tree at home ... Tropical plant, the Annona muricata appreciates the sun and heat, and must be protected from frost in our latitudes, ideally in greenhouse shelter. Be sure to be patient: seed germination takes 15 to 60 days, and fruits, if they deign to appear, do so three to four years after

planting!

9 781723 735257